W9-BNR-311

A Woman's Guide to
Personal Safety

A Woman's Guide to Personal Safety

By Janeé Harteau and Holly Keegel

Fairview Press   Minneapolis

Library of Congress Cataloging-in-Publication Data
Harteau, Janeé, 1964–
        A woman's guide to personal safety / by
    Janeé Harteau and Holly Keegel.
            p.   cm.
        ISBN 1-57749-065-7 (pbk. : alk. paper)
        1. Women--Crimes against--United States--Prevention. 2. Self-defense for women. 3. Safety education--United States. 4. Rape--United States--Prevention.   5. Wife Abuse--United States--Prevention.   I. Keegel, Holly, 1964–   . II. Title.
    HV6250.4.W65H38   1998
    613.6'6'082--dc21   97-466389
                                                                    CIP

First Printing: March 1998
Printed in the United States of America
02 01 00 99 98   7 6 5 4 3 2 1

Cover design: Laurie Duren

Fairview Press publications, including *A Woman's Guide to Personal Safety,* do not necessarily reflect the philosophy of Fairview Healthcare Services.

CONTENTS

We would like to dedicate this book to the two strongest, most influential women we know.

Our mothers.

INTRODUCTION

As police officers, we have responded to a number of crimes against women. Arresting the perpetrators has given us insight into how attackers choose their victims.

As women, we have been victims of crime. We, too, know what it is like to feel vulnerable.

According to the 1996 National Crime Victimization Survey, more than two-and-a-half million women in the United States experience violence each year.

Violence against women is a tremendous problem in this country. Women, however, are responding to the challenge—they are learning to make their safety a priority.

Our goal is to help prevent women from becoming victims. It is not always possible to avoid a dangerous situation. But there are ways to minimize your risks and, in many cases, avoid becoming a victim altogether.

Too many women live their lives in fear—an unhealthy, and frequently unnecessary, condition. The information on the following pages is intended to help you build confidence in your ability to protect yourself.

There is no reason to walk around feeling afraid all the time. If a dangerous situation arises, you will be prepared to respond to it. You are your own best defense against crime.

SAFETY TIPS

How Attackers
Choose Their Victims

Most attackers look for individuals who are:

- Women

- Elderly

- Mentally or physically challenged

- Alone

- Distracted or inattentive

- Unlikely to put up a fight

How Attackers Choose Their Victims

Attackers also watch for opportunities:

- A stranded motorist
- A broken window
- A dark parking lot
- A dangling purse
- An unlocked door
- An open garage

How Attackers Choose Their Victims

It is unfortunate that women must live with the threat of being attacked. After all, we're not the ones who are committing these crimes. Why should we have to change our behaviors to be safe?

It isn't fair, but it is a reality we must face.

Be prepared for anything. This is the first and most important step in assuring your safety.

If you don't act like a victim, you are less likely to become one. Keep in mind the following tips.

Be Alert

Know your surroundings.

Be assertive.

Walk with confidence.

Observe the people around you.

Know where you are going.

Use eye contact. Don't look down or away, but don't invite a confrontation by staring.

Sixth Sense

Listen to it. Trust it. Use it.

Awareness is the key to preventing a dangerous situation.

If something feels wrong or out of place, it probably is.

Always trust your intuition.

Have a Plan

Suspects have a plan. You should, too.

If you were attacked, what would you do? Have you thought about it?

Would you fight? Freeze up? Run away?

If someone tried to kidnap, rape, or kill you, could you fight back?

It is unpleasant to think about, but you will be better prepared to defend yourself if you know your capabilities.

Imagine that the worst has happened— someone is trying to rape or kill you.

Have a Plan

Envision yourself fighting back with everything you've got.

Imagine what you would have to do to get away. Aim for the eyes, nose, windpipe. Use your teeth, fingers, fists, legs, knees. Feel your strength. Remember, your life may be at stake.

Having a plan is the key to minimizing a dangerous situation—and possibly avoiding it all together.

Rehearse your plan. Repetition will make your reaction to a dangerous situation seem like a natural response.

Have an Escape

In strange or unfamiliar places, make it a habit to take a mental note of your surroundings. Identify all avenues of escape and look for people who can help you if you are attacked.

Look for:
- Doors
- Elevators
- Windows
- Stairways
- Any opportunity to get away on foot, by car, or by bicycle

Have an Escape

By knowing where the exits are ahead of time, you will gain extra seconds that could save your life.

If your plan is to distract your attacker and run, envision yourself running away, using these exits to escape.

Practice finding an escape at your office, a friend's or neighbor's house, the parking lot at the mall, and in your car. Think to yourself, "If I were attacked right here, right now, what could I do to protect myself? How could I keep myself safe?"

Don't Panic

Have a plan and put it into action.

Don't freeze up.

Use your rush of adrenaline to give you the strength to get away.

Distract the Attacker

Always try to keep a barrier—like a vehicle or shopping cart—between you and your attacker.

Scream, kick, push, shove—do anything you can to distract or distance yourself from the attacker so you can get away safely.

Report All Crimes

If you are the victim of a crime, no matter how small, report it.

You may just prevent another woman from becoming a victim.

CALLING 911

To report a crime, suspicious activity in your neighborhood, or a medical emergency, dial 911 on your telephone.

This will connect you to a dispatcher, who will send a squad car or ambulance immediately.

The dispatcher will probably keep you on the phone while remaining in constant communication with the police or emergency medical services.

He or she will update them on any changes in your situation.

In the meantime, the dispatcher will ask you a number of questions that may or may not seem related to your situation.

He or she will tell you how to administer first aid, if it is necessary.

Otherwise, the dispatcher will try to keep you calm and focused until help arrives.

A common misconception is that the longer you stay on the phone with the dispatcher, the longer it takes for the police or ambulance to reach you.

The fact is, it makes no difference how long the dispatcher keeps you on the phone. When a crime or medical emergency is in progress, help is already on the way.

Try to remain on the phone with the dispatcher. Circumstances may change in a matter of seconds, and you will need to relay any new information.

Calling 911: A Scenario

You are alone in your house watching television when you hear glass shatter in the kitchen.

You immediately dial 911 on your cellular phone. The police are on their way.

You tell the dispatcher that you hear someone crawling through the kitchen window. The dispatcher informs the police.

Remembering your safety plan, you run out of the house, taking the cellular phone with you.

On your way to the front door, you see a man wearing a black knit cap and black clothing walk toward the living room. Once outside, you relay this information to the dispatcher, who again updates the police officers.

The dispatcher tells you that the squad car has arrived, and the police pull up to your house. The man runs out the back door.

Because you were able to give the dispatcher a description of the man, he is caught by another police officer down the block.

DESCRIBING YOUR ATTACKER

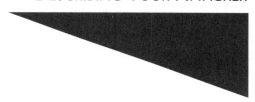

If you are attacked, an accurate and detailed description is the most important information you can give the police. Describe your attacker from head to toe. Note:

- Sex, race, and age.

- Height and weight. Use yourself, a doorway, or a fixed object to judge the attacker's height.

- Hair color, length, and style (curly, wavy, straight, or balding). Also note if the hair was dirty, greasy, or unkempt.

- Facial hair (clean shaven, un-shaven, or having a beard, mustache, or goatee).

- Eye color, and whether the attacker wore glasses.

- Jewelry, such as earrings, unique chains, and rings.

- Clothing. Be as detailed and descriptive as possible. Note color, style, and brand names, including emblems and logos. Describe the length of the attacker's coat or jacket (full, waist, or knee length).

Most crimes happen in a very short period of time, and it can be difficult to get a detailed description.

Try to focus on unusual characteristics, such as missing, crooked, or decayed teeth; scars; birthmarks; tattoos; deformities; a pock-marked or bad complexion; an unusual odor or tone of voice— anything that might make your attacker stand out.

If your attacker carried a weapon, try to describe it to the police.

If you saw a gun, for example, note if it was a revolver (which has a cylinder) or a semi-automatic (which has a magazine and a clip).

If the attacker had a knife, describe what kind of knife (kitchen, utility, pocket, or hunting knife), and the length of the blade.

A Detailed Description

The attacker was a white male, sixteen to twenty years old, approximately 5'10" tall, with a thin build. He had greasy, straight brown hair of medium length. He was unshaven, wore a white t-shirt with blue stripes, and had a tattoo on his right upper arm. He was armed with a kitchen knife with a wooden handle. He left in a blue pick-up truck with several bumper stickers on the rear. He drove north through the alley.

STAYING SAFE IN
DANGEROUS SITUATIONS

CARJACKING

Between 1987 and 1992, an average of 35,000 carjackings were attempted each year. Carjackers succeeded in stealing the vehicle 52% of the time. A weapon was used 77% of the time.

(U.S. Department of Justice, 1994)

Keep your car doors locked, especially when you are inside.

When approaching your car, always have your keys in your hand and ready for use. If you need to, you can use your keys as a weapon.

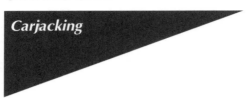

Carjacking

In dark or poorly-lighted parking lots, try to avoid walking to your car alone.

If security is available, ask them to escort you.

When walking toward your car, look around to be sure no one is following you or lurking near your vehicle.

In a parking lot or ramp, walk down the center of the driveway. Never walk next to parked vehicles—someone may be hiding there, ready to jump out and grab you.

Attacks on women often occur after someone has broken into a vehicle and hidden inside.

Check for broken windows and glass fragments in and around your car.

Always look in the backseat and other passenger areas before getting into the vehicle.

If you see someone inside your car, walk away from the vehicle immediately and get help. Try to act casual to avoid alerting the attacker.

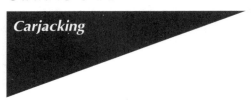

Carjacking

If you are approached by an attacker outside of your car:

- Yell, scream, do what you can to call attention to yourself.

- Never get inside the car with the attacker.

If an attacker wants you to come with him or her, he or she wants more than your car and plans to hurt you, possibly even kill you.

Carjacking

If an attacker is armed with a weapon and demands your vehicle, let him or her take it.

Never put yourself at risk just to save your property.

Your goal is to get away safely. Let the police catch the attacker.

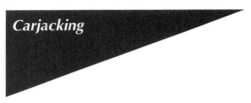

Carjacking

Once inside your vehicle:

- Make sure that all the doors are locked and the windows are rolled up.

- If an attacker is present, honk your horn repeatedly to alert security and passersby.

- Drive away immediately.

If an attacker stands in your way and tries to keep you from leaving, don't stop the car—run over him or her if you have to.

If a Carjacker Steals
Your Vehicle

Notify the police immediately.

Know the make, model, year, color, and license plate number of your vehicle.

If your car has any damage, markings, or unique features, tell the police. This may help them recover the car, especially if the license plates have been changed.

If a Carjacker Steals Your Vehicle

Note the direction in which the carjacker drove.

Give officers a detailed description of the carjacker, including the type of weapon, if one was used.

If the carjacker said he or she had a gun, tell the police, even if you never saw one.

SEXUAL ASSAULT

In the United States, 1.3 women are raped every minute.

(National Victim Center, 1992)

It is estimated that one out of every three American women will be sexually assaulted in her lifetime.

(National Victim Center, 1992)

Four out of five women who fight their attackers are able to get away.

(National Center for the Prevention and Control of Rape, 1992)

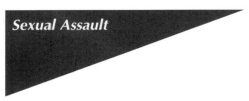

Sexual Assault

Sexual assault might be committed by a stranger, an acquaintance, a friend—even a boyfriend or husband.

In fact, victims frequently know their attacker.

If you or someone you know has been sexually assaulted, call 1-800-656-HOPE to get in touch with your local counseling center.

Outdoors

One out of every four rapes takes place
in a public area or in a parking lot.
(U.S. Department of Justice, 1994)

No one should feel compelled to stay
indoors out of fear of being attacked.

This would be unrealistic—and unfair.

But the threat of sexual assault is a reality that women face. You will be better
able to protect yourself against an outdoor attack by following some basic
safety tips.

Outdoor Sexual Assault

Do not walk or jog alone at night.

Stay in populated areas with good lighting.

Do not wear headphones—you may not be able to hear if someone approaches you from behind, and you will appear vulnerable to an attacker.

If you do wear headphones, keep the music low enough to hear what is going on around you.

Outdoor Sexual Assault

Change your routes and workout times frequently. Some attackers will watch their victims for weeks to learn their patterns before assaulting them.

Always be alert. Prepare yourself for a dangerous situation. Look for avenues of escape and rehearse your safety plan.

Wear comfortable shoes when walking outdoors, even when walking from your car to your workplace. If you must bring dress shoes, carry them in a bag and put them on at work.

Outdoor Sexual Assault

If someone approaches you and you feel uncomfortable, cross the street or change your direction.

Many attackers approach their victims on the pretense of striking up a conversation or seeking assistance. If someone stops to ask you questions, don't get distracted. Just keep moving.

Often a woman's natural response is to be polite, even when faced with a potentially dangerous situation. There is no need to be polite. If you feel threatened, make your feelings known.

Outdoor Sexual Assault

For example, if you feel uncomfortable when a stranger stops to ask for directions, do not answer. Keep walking.

If the stranger persists and tries to stop you from leaving, say, "I have somewhere I need to be," and walk away.

If this doesn't work, say, "Leave me alone." Be firm and don't back down.

If you continue walking or tell the stranger to leave you alone, this should be the end of it.

Outdoor Sexual Assault

If the threat does not go away, however, or if it escalates, so should your response.

You may need to distract the stranger. Protest loudly to bring attention to yourself or yell for someone to call the police. Look for an escape and put your safety plan into action.

Do whatever it takes to remove yourself from danger. Your instincts will guide you.

There is no need to apologize for your behavior. Remember, you don't have to be nice to strangers. Nice can be used against you.

In Your Home

Nearly six out of ten sexual assaults occur in the victim's home or the home of a friend, relative, or neighbor.
(U.S. Department of Justice, 1997)

We tend to think of home as a place of safety and security.

The fact is, many assaults happen to women in their own homes.

Be prepared to defend yourself.

Keep your doors and windows locked, especially on the ground level, and especially at night.

**Sexual Assault
in Your Home**

If you have a weapon or self-defense device, be sure to keep it within reach and ready for use.

Keep a telephone close to your bed, preferably a cordless or cellular phone, so you can go outside or move from room to room.

A cellular telephone is best—if a phone is taken off the hook in another room, you will still be able to dial 911.

**Sexual Assault
in Your Home**

If you hear a strange noise outside, call the police immediately. This way, the police will already by on their way if someone should get inside.

If someone breaks into your home, GET OUT.

Don't panic.

Remember the safety plans you have learned and practiced.

**Sexual Assault
in Your Home**

If you are unable to get out, grab the telephone and lock yourself in a room.

Call the police and stay on the line with the dispatcher until they arrive.

If you are alone, call out to a husband, friend, or boyfriend to make the intruder believe someone else is in the house with you.

**Sexual Assault
in Your Home**

Always look for an opportunity to escape.

If the attacker catches you, you will have to decide whether or not to resist. Trust your intuition—you will know what to do.

Most attackers have a certain plan or pattern. If you break their pattern for a moment, they may be caught off guard, giving you time to escape.

**Sexual Assault
in Your Home**

Screaming, shoving, or kicking may distract your attacker long enough for you to get away.

Vomiting, gagging, defecating, or urinating may help stop a potential rape. If you choose to fight, give it your all. Don't hold back—find the strength to win.

Remember, women have a lot of strength in their legs and lower body.

**Sexual Assault
in Your Home**

If you choose not to fight or you cannot get away, use the power of your mind.

Memorize every inch of your attacker. Create a mental picture so you can provide a detailed description to the police.

Do whatever it takes to stay alive.

Don't give up—your survival may depend on it.

Once your attacker has left, telephone the police immediately.

Acquaintance Rape

In nearly three out of four sexual assaults, the victim knew her attacker.
(U.S. Department of Justice, 1997)

"No" means "no," whether it is your boss, a friend, your boyfriend, or your husband.

Other than the fact that you know your attacker, there is no difference between a date rape and a stranger rape. Still, there are steps you can take to help prevent an attack.

When you go out on a first date, give a friend or family member your date's full name, address, phone number, and other important information.

Acquaintance Rape

Bring along cash for a taxi and enough change for emergency phone calls.

Try to go to a public place, or arrange to meet your date somewhere well populated. If possible, drive yourself so you can leave if you feel uncomfortable.

Avoid drinking too much alcohol. If you find yourself in a dangerous or uncomfortable situation, you want to be fully in control.

Acquaintance Rape

If you are attacked, put your safety plan into action. Don't hold back, even if you consider the attacker your friend.

Do whatever you can to survive the attack.

Get away as soon as you feel the time is right and notify the police.

Date Rape Drugs

"Roofies," GHB, and other date rape drugs are becoming more widespread. Many are tasteless, colorless, odorless— and sometimes fatal.

A rapist will dissolve these chemicals in a woman's drink, wait for her to black out, and then rape her. When the woman wakes up the next morning, she frequently has no recollection of the night before.

Do not allow your date to bring you your drink. Get your own drinks, and never leave them unattended.

If You Are Sexually Assaulted

Do not bathe or shower.

It is extremely important for rape sur-
vivors to go to the hospital for medical
treatment and a special exam.

If you bathe or shower, you will wash
away the proof that you have been raped,
which police will need to catch your
attacker. Let a doctor examine you first.

If You Are Sexually Assaulted

Call the police immediately.

Do not move or touch anything connected with your attacker.

Do not dispose of clothing, sheets, or condoms. These items are evidence, and it is crucial not to contaminate them.

If You Are Sexually Assaulted

As soon as you can, write down every-thing you can remember about your attacker while it is fresh in your mind.

Write down a physical description, includ-ing scars, tattoos, tone of voice, and odor.

Note everything your attacker may have touched or left fingerprints on.

Tell the police everything the attacker said and did, and point out every part of the home he was in. This will help the police when they are collecting evidence.

If You Are Sexually Assaulted

Some attackers learn about their victims by burglarizing them, then they return at a later date to assault them. If your home was burglarized recently, share this information with the police.

A sexual assault is a traumatic event. It is important to surround yourself with people who will comfort and support you through the weeks and months to come.

CAMPUS SAFETY

It is estimated that one in every four college women has suffered a rape or attempted rape.

(National Victim Center, 1992)

Sexual assault, including acquaintance rape, is a growing problem on college campuses. Again, women must use caution and learn how to protect themselves.

When visiting or moving to a college campus, inquire about escorts and other rape prevention services.

Do not put yourself in a potentially dangerous situation.

Campus Safety

Keep in mind that alcohol or drugs can make you vulnerable to an attack.

Do not allow yourself to become so intoxicated that you are unable to care for yourself or recall the evening's events the next day.

Use good judgment at fraternity and sorority parties.

The use of date rape drugs is on the rise, particularly on college campuses. Never accept an open drink at a party. Instead, choose a closed can of beer or soda, and never leave it unattended.

Campus Safety

Don't go anywhere with someone you do nct know well.

Be careful about letting other people into your room late at night, even if you know them.

When going on a first date, it is best not to go alone. Double date, or go some-place where there will be other people around. Make sure that a close friend or family member knows who you are with. Give them your date's address and phone number.

Campus Safety

Avoid walking alone or going places by yourself, especially after dark. The more people you are with, the less likely it is that an assault will occur.

Carry your backpack securely in front of you. If you carry it on both shoulders, an attacker could grab the pack to keep you from escaping. If your backpack hangs off one shoulder, you may be injured if someone tries to steal it from you. By holding your backpack tightly in front of you, you will deter a thief, but remain mobile enough to escape a dangerous situation.

Campus Safety

Take routes that are well-lighted and populated with other students.

If you think you are being followed, go inside the nearest business and wait until the individual has passed before you continue walking.

If the individual follows you inside, notify an employee and call campus security or the police.

Report all crimes that occur on campus. Criminals continue to commit crimes if their victims don't make a report.

DOMESTIC VIOLENCE

Nearly two out of every three female victims of violence were related to or knew their attackers.

> (National Crime Victimization Survey, 1996)

A domestic assault occurs once every nine seconds in the United States.

> (FBI Uniform Crime Report, 1996)

Forty-two percent of all female murder victims are killed by their current or former husband, boyfriend, or partner.

> (Family Violence Prevention Fund, 1990)

Domestic Violence

Domestic violence:

- Is a serious crime

- Is never the survivor's fault

- Leads to serious injury or death

- Affects everyone, especially children

If it happens once, it will happen again. Nothing you can do will change that.

If you or someone you know is a victim of domestic violence, call 1-800-END-ABUSE.

Domestic Violence

If you are hit, bit, pushed, kicked, choked, raped, or otherwise injured by your partner, or if your partner threatens to kill you:

- Notify the police immediately, even if it has never happened before.
- Get proper medical treatment.
- Take photographs of your injuries.
- Complete all the police reports. Police reports will help document the abuse, and documentation will help if you decide to prosecute or file for a restraining order.
- Prosecute. The abuse will not stop without help.

Domestic Violence

Be strong.

Remove yourself and your children from the danger.

Take back control of your life.

Contact your local domestic violence shelter. Volunteers will support you in deciding whether to leave the relationship, and when.

You don't have to tell your partner that you are leaving.

Domestic Violence

Have a safety plan. Gather the essentials:
- Money, checks, and credit cards
- Driver's license, green card
- Important phone numbers
- Extra set of car keys
- Spare clothes
- Prescription drugs
- Spare eye glasses or contact lenses
- Birth certificates and social security numbers for you and your children
- Anything else you might need

Domestic Violence

Hide these in one place or leave them with a trusted neighbor so your partner can't find them.

If you think you might be in danger, take these items and GET OUT.

Remember, your partner can't hurt you if he or she can't find you.

Restraining Orders

If you are a victim of domestic violence, know your legal rights. Call your local shelter, abuse hotline, or attorney's office for information.

In most states, a victim has the option to file for a restraining order if certain criteria are met.

A restraining order is a legal document, signed by a judge, which prohibits any contact between the victim and the abuser.

An abuser who violates a restraining order may be arrested.

Restraining Orders

The purpose of a restraining order is to give police the authority to arrest an abuser just for making contact with the victim.

The victim does not have to wait until she is threatened or injured before getting assistance.

A restraining order might help keep an abuser away, but it does not guarantee your safety. Do not allow yourself to feel safe simply because you have a restraining order. It is a false sense of security that could leave you more vulnerable to attack.

Restraining Orders

After all, if someone really wants to hurt you, a restraining order probably won't stop him or her from trying.

If you choose to get a restraining order, don't let down your guard. Keep your crime prevention strategies in place and make safety your number one priority.

Some victims think that getting a restraining order will enrage their abuser, increasing the likelihood of an attack. This is not the case. The threat of going to jail may keep an abuser away, or it will have no effect whatsoever, but it will not cause an abuser to become more violent.

Restraining Orders

If you think your abuser will be undeterred by a restraining order, consider getting one anyway. If he or she even tries to contact you, police may be able to intervene.

If you have a restraining order, do not call or invite your abuser to your home, no matter how much you love him or her.

It would be unethical to coerce your abuser into violating a restraining order. More importantly, you would be risking your safety.

STALKING

It is estimated that as many as 200,000 American women are currently being stalked, and one in twenty women will become targets of stalking behavior at least once during their lifetime.

(National Victim Center, 1993)

Stalking is such a common problem that many women do not take it seriously until it is too late.

It may look like "persistence," at first— frequent, harmless attention. You might be nice to this individual and try to let him or her down easy, but the problem only seems to escalate.

Stalking

In other cases, stalking shows itself for what it is: blatant harassment. You might feel threatened from the start. Your stalker's actions may become more and more drastic and unnerving over time.

Stalking is a serious crime that sometimes leads to assault, even murder.

If someone follows you, calls you repeatedly, or persistently pays you unwelcome attention, notify the police.

If you know your stalker or think you are being stalked for a reason, share this information with the authorities as well.

Stalking

Fill out police reports and consider filing for a restraining order. If you take swift legal action, you may be able to defuse the situation before anybody gets hurt.

Do not respond to your stalker's letters or phone calls. This would only encourage the stalker.

Keep a record of your stalker's behavior. Each time he or she calls, writes, or follows you, note the time and date.

In the meantime, remain aware of your surroundings and be prepared to put your safety plan into action.

THE INTERNET

Computer use is on the rise, and many women are meeting people—and sometimes dating—over the Internet. Naturally, there are some safety issues to consider when using this new technology.

Don't believe everything you read.

To avoid harassment in a chat room, consider using a male name or nickname.

When talking or corresponding with people on-line, always remember that they are strangers.

The Internet

Do not give anyone your full name, address, credit card number, or other personal information (unless you are dealing with a legitimate business on a secure site).

If you decide to meet an Internet acquaintance in person, meet him or her in a location you are familiar with. Do not meet this person alone. Go to a public place, and bring someone with you.

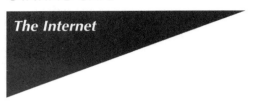

The Internet

If you list your name on an Internet registration site, be aware that the information you enter will be available to others. If someone wants to find you, he or she could use your name and address to print out a map that highlights your location in your neighborhood.

If an Internet provider calls you on the telephone, make sure the caller is legitimate before answering any personal questions. Ask for his or her full name and the main phone number to the office. Then, hang up, call the office, and ask to be connected to this individual.

If You Are Harassed
on the Internet

Tell the harasser that his or her e-mail, posts, or comments are not welcome, and that you want him or her to stop immediately.

Contact the site administrator to report the problem. Write to postmaster@[site name].com, or you can find the address on the Web by looking up the site name (through Yahoo or AltaVista, for example).

Ask the site administrator to ban the harasser from the site if the problem continues.

WORK SAFETY

Each year, nearly one million people in the United States become victims of violent crime while working or on duty.

(U.S. Department of Labor, 1996)

The workplace is the scene of 8% of all rapes and 16% of all assaults.

(*The Economist,* 1994)

Homicide is the leading cause of death in the workplace for women.

(National Institute for Occupational Safety and Health, 1996)

In the Office

Your safety at work is just as crucial as your safety at home, outdoors, and in the car. As always, you need to use caution and remain aware of your surroundings.

If you manage a business, designate a main entrance for visitors and delivery personnel to check in. Issue visitor passes so you know who is coming and going.

Keep all entrances to the building well-lighted, and make sure the business name and address are visible. Good lighting will not only appeal to customers and workers, it will deter many criminals.

In the Office

Familiarize yourself with your workplace. Learn all of the exits and be aware of blind corners.

Know the exact address of your office so emergency personnel will be able to respond quickly to a crisis.

Get acquainted with fellow employees so you know who is allowed access to your workplace.

Ask security to escort you to and from your car, especially at night.

If security officers aren't available, walk with a group or another coworker.

If you are working alone, make sure you tell someone. Check in with this person from time to time to let him or her know that you are okay.

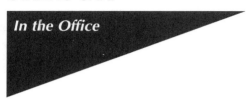

In the Office

Never leave your purse, wallet, check-book, credit cards, or other personal items unattended. Take them with you or lock them in a secure place, even when visiting a coworker or making a quick trip to the restroom.

A thief will often enter a business as a customer, client, or employee. If the business is not monitored, the thief will have plenty of time to move from office to office.

In the Office

Remember, many thieves are smooth talkers who can play the part of a customer or client.

Use your intuition. If something feels wrong, it probably is. Report suspicious activity to the management or police.

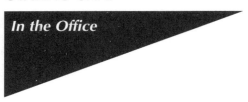

In the Office

Look for potential attackers who might be hanging around restrooms, elevators, stairways, parking lots, entrances, and exits.

If an unfamiliar person appears to be lurking around the office, get a good description of the individual and inform the management, security, or police.

If another employee is threatening, harassing, or following you, be sure to tell someone and make a police report. Take these incidents seriously, even if the harasser is someone you know.

If a current or former boyfriend, husband, partner, or family member has been threatening you, it is important to tell someone at work. Domestic violence attacks and murders frequently occur in the workplace.

Don't confront these individuals, especially if they are angry. Let the police handle it.

Out of the Office

Caregivers, contractors, builders, decorators, salespeople, tutors, housekeepers, UPS workers, repair people, social service workers, and post office workers are just a few of the professionals who visit private residences in the course of their work.

If you do business in unfamiliar houses and neighborhoods, there are important safety tips you ought to keep in mind.

Out of the Office

Before making your visit, get a little background information. Talk to employees who have visited the house before. If the house is in a high crime area, you may want to contact the local police for information.

Find out how many people will be at the house you intend to visit.

Always notify your office or a family member when making a home visit. Give them the name and address of the person you are meeting, as well as the time that you expect to return. Call them as soon as you arrive, then call again when you leave.

Out of the Office

Know where you are going, especially in unfamiliar neighborhoods. If you can, drive by the area prior to your visit.

Bring written directions.

Do not pull over and ask for assistance in a residential area. You are more vulnerable if you appear lost.

Carry a cellular phone with you at all times.

If you don't have a cellular phone, always know the location of the nearest pay phone.

Out of the Office

If possible, make your visit in the daytime. Daylight will allow you to see everything around you, and there will be more people nearby if something should happen.

If you have to make a night visit, try to bring another person with you. Otherwise, call someone when you get to the house and let them know when you expect to leave.

As you drive through the neighborhood, keep an eye out for businesses and other safe places so you know where you can go if you encounter a problem.

Out of the Office

If a group of unfamiliar people are loitering near the house when you arrive, and you feel uncomfortable, don't go inside. Leave and return again after a few minutes. If the people are still there, come back at another time.

When you get to the door, take a few seconds to listen inside. If you hear yelling or fighting, there may be an assault in progress. Don't jeopardize your safety. Leave immediately and notify the police.

Out of the Office

Once inside the house, scan the area to make sure you are safe.

If you see things that make you feel uncomfortable, such as knives or other weapons, ask that they be put in another room.

Try to sit near an exit, so you can leave in a hurry if you have to.

It is always appropriate to leave and come back another time.

Out of the Office

If anyone in the house appears intoxi-cated or on drugs, or if a fight breaks out, don't become confrontational.

Tell them this is not a good time and you will come back later.

Always remain in control of your visit. If a situation doesn't feel right, it is better to come back on a safer occasion.

Burglary

A burglary takes place every thirteen seconds in the United States.
  (FBI Uniform Crime Report, 1996)

In two-thirds of the burglaries in 1995, the burglar gained entry through an unlocked door or open window.
  (Bureau of Justice Statistics, 1995)

It's a good idea to keep a written record of your valuables—with brand names, model numbers, and serial numbers—in a safe place, such as with a trusted friend or relative. If you are burglarized, this information may help the police recover your belongings.

Burglary

Don't leave purses, checkbooks, credit cards, cash, or jewelry where they can be seen through the window.

Make it difficult for a burglar to break into your home. Burglars are looking for easy access and do not want a confrontation.

Get a dog. Most burglars are afraid of dogs and usually won't target houses that have them.

Burglary

Keep doors and windows locked, even when you are home. Burglars have been known to enter through an unlocked front door while residents were in their backyard.

Secure all doors with a good lock, such as a deadbolt.

Install a large strike plate with long screws on the frame of the door. This can help prevent a burglar from forcing the door open.

Burglary

Secure all windows.

If you have older locks, such as "clamshells," buy pegs or adjustable locks from the hardware store and attach them to your window frames. These will allow windows to open only partially, preventing a burglar from getting inside. The windows can be opened all the way in an emergency.

Basement windows often mean easy access for burglars. Install adjustable locks on the windows or put up bars on the outside.

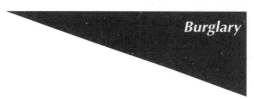

Sliding glass doors are easy to remove from their tracks. Keep these doors locked. For extra protection, install a "charlie" bar, which goes across the middle of the door, or find a long pole to fit inside the entire length of the track.

Set automatic lights to go off inside your home when you are away. Change the times frequently.

Vary the times that you come and go, so burglars do not learn your schedule.

Burglary

Install an alarm system. Find a well-established alarm company that will help you choose a system that fits your lifestyle. Some motion alarms do not work well with pets, for example.

If you are looking for a new home, choose a neighborhood with adequate street lights.

Use motion lights on the outside of your house.

Burglary

Keep trees and bushes trimmed so they don't block windows or doors. Burglars look for entrances that are partially hidden from view, giving them more time to break in.

Make sure your house numbers are visible and large enough for emergency personnel to find you quickly.

If you come home to a broken or open door or window, do not go inside. Go to a neighbor's house or nearby phone and call the police. Let the police check to see if the burglars are still inside your house.

Burglary

Join a block club or neighborhood watch group. These organizations not only give you an opportunity to get to know your neighbors, they help make your neighborhood a safe place to live.

If your neighborhood doesn't already have a block club or watch group, contact your local police department for information on how to start one.

If Your House Is Burglarized

Telephone the police immediately.

Do not touch anything.

Give the police a complete list of the items that were taken. Include name brands, models, and serial numbers.

If checks or credit cards were stolen, call your bank or credit card company to notify them of the theft.

If Your House Is Burglarized

Report any guns that were taken from your house. Be sure to tell police the models and serial numbers.

It is not uncommon for a burglar to return to the same house and steal again. To avoid another burglary, repair broken windows and doors as soon as possible.

Apartment Safety

Avoid renting a ground-floor apartment, especially one with a sliding glass door.

Choose an apartment with on-site security and gated or underground parking.

If you have an underground parking area, look in your rearview mirror after you pull in and wait until the garage door closes to make sure no one walks in behind you.

STAYING SAFE

Apartment Safety

When walking to your apartment door, have the key in your hand and ready for use.

Do not tell strangers or acquaintances that you live alone.

Do not open the door for strangers or solicitors.

Never let strangers use your telephone. If they have an emergency, you can call the police for them.

Apartment Safety

Do not buzz in strangers or allow non-residents to walk inside behind you.

If you notice strangers loitering in or around the building, notify management, security, or the police.

Do not use the laundry room, exercise room, or other facilities late at night or when no one else is around.

If you are having repairs or deliveries made, schedule a specific time so you can be at home when the workers arrive.

Apartment Safety

Although caretakers have a right to enter your apartment for repairs and deliveries, limit their access.

If they seem to be inside your home too often when you are away, notify the management.

Make sure you have good locks on your doors and windows.

Hang blinds or shades on your windows, especially in the bedroom.

Do not list your full name on the mailbox, buzzer, or in the phone book. Use your first initial and last name, so a burglar will not be able to tell if you are male or female.

Use automatic lights when you are not home, and vary the times they go on.

Attackers often watch their victims for weeks before they attack, so change your routines. Try to come and go at different times. Vary the routes you take to work, to the grocery store, and to walk the dog.

THEFT

A theft occurs every four seconds in the United States.

(FBI Uniform Crime Report, 1996)

Like many crimes, theft takes less than a minute to commit.

Most thefts occur at random, when an opportunity arises, and can usually be prevented through common sense.

Report all thefts. This may prevent someone else from becoming a victim.

Theft

Keep your garage door closed, even when you are home. An open garage is an invitation to take bicycles, lawn mowers, snowblowers, tools, and anything else you might value.

Keep doors and windows locked when you leave, even if you are just going in the backyard for a few minutes or making a quick trip to the store.

Staying Safe

When attending concerts, fairs, and other events that attract large crowds, carry your cash and valuables in your front pocket or a fanny pack.

If someone bumps into you in a large crowd, immediately check your purse and pockets to be sure that nothing is missing.

Never leave your purse or wallet unattended in a public place, not even while you use the phone or restroom for a moment.

Mailbox theft is common, especially during the first few days of the month when many people receive welfare checks and other federal payments in the mail.

If you are expecting a check (or a box of blank checks) in the mail, and it does not arrive within a reasonable length of time, call the company or bank to see when it was sent.

Theft

Never give strangers personal information over the phone, unless they call from a company you do business with and they ask appropriate questions.

If you want to be sure that a caller is phoning from a legitimate company, ask for his or her name and the company's general phone number. Tell the caller that you will call the general phone number and ask to be connected to him or her in a few minutes.

If you receive a letter or telephone call stating that you have won something, never send money or give out a social security or credit card number to collect the prize.

Always ask questions to check on the validity of a business.

If you are not interested in what they are selling or it sounds "fishy," hang up.

Never feel pressured to listen to strangers or participate in a conversation that makes you uncomfortable.

AUTO THEFT

A vehicle is stolen ever 23 seconds in the United States.
(FBI Uniform Crime Report, 1996)

It's no fun going out to your car and not finding it. You can save yourself a lot of money and hassle by following some basic guidelines.

Lock your vehicle doors, even when your car is parked in your driveway or garage.

Always lock your garage doors.

Auto Theft

Never leave personal belongings visible inside your vehicle, including purses, wallets, checkbooks, credit cards, cellular phones, sports equipment, briefcases, gifts, lap top computers, or camera equipment.

Try to park your car in a populated area, under streetlights, and near other vehicles.

Avoid parking in dark or secluded areas that could allow a thief to hide while breaking into your car.

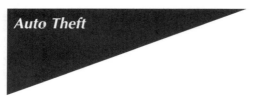

Auto Theft

If you have packages or other valuables that should be secured, try to lock them in the trunk without being seen.

If your vehicle doesn't already have an alarm system, have one put in.

For extra protection, install an anti-theft device that will lock the steering column.

Never keep your vehicle running or leave your keys in the ignition while you warm up the car or run into a convenience store.

Purse Snatching

Purse snatching is a crime of opportunity. If you don't carry a purse, it cannot be taken from you.

If you choose to carry a purse, don't use shoulder straps. A clutch purse is much more difficult for a purse snatcher to grab.

If you carry a purse with shoulder straps, hold it under your coat or close to your body and keep a tight grip on it at all times.

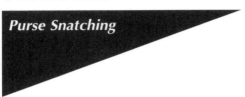

Purse Snatching

Never wear the straps diagonally across your body or twisted around your wrist. If someone grabs the purse and runs, the straps may injure your neck or arm.

Prepare for your day—bring only one check or credit card, along with a small amount of cash.

Carry your keys in your hand. This prevents a purse snatcher from taking your keys from the purse and using them to burglarize your house later.

Never hang your purse on a chair or leave it unattended in a public place.

If Your Purse Is Stolen

Notify the police or security immediately.

Describe the purse snatcher in detail.

Note if he or she escaped on foot, with a bicycle, or in a car.

If the purse snatcher drove off in a car, give police a detailed description of the vehicle. Include the make, model, year, color, and license plate number.

If Your Purse Is Stolen

Even if you get a partial license plate number or notice only that the car is from out of state, share this information with the police.

Note the direction in which the purse snatcher escaped. This will help the police locate him or her more quickly.

Report missing checks and credits cards to the appropriate agencies so the purse snatcher can't use them.

If Your Purse Is Stolen

Purse snatchers are looking for quick cash. They will usually take the money and discard the purse.

Look for your purse in nearby dumpsters and garbage cans, under bushes, and in yards.

The money will be gone, but you will probably recover items that would be harder to replace, such as a driver's license or social security card.

ATMs

There have been several instances where individuals have been beaten—and sometimes murdered—while withdrawing their money from an automated teller machine.

Fortunately, attacks like these can often be avoided if you take the proper precautions.

If you feel unsafe at anytime, LEAVE. It isn't worth losing your life over a few dollars.

Do not use an ATM alone at night.

If you see a stranger lurking near the ATM or in the parking lot, either wait until the individual leaves or find another machine.

Report suspicious behavior.

Don't dig for your card in your purse or wallet—have the card ready when you approach the ATM.

Leave your purse at home or in the car.

ATMs

Do not count your money in front of other people. When the money comes out of the machine, take it quickly and put it in your front pants pocket.

Once you return to your vehicle, lock the doors. Do not hang around the parking lot.

If you are using a drive-through ATM, keep your doors locked and your windows rolled up. Have your card ready.

ATMs

Roll down your driver-side window, complete your transaction quickly, and roll the window up again.

If another car appears to be lingering in the parking lot, drive to a different ATM.

If you think you are being followed, drive to a police station, fire station, or place of business.

Public Transportation

When you take the same bus or subway to work everyday, it is easy to fall into a false sense of security.

Remember, having other commuters around you does not make you less vulnerable.

If you travel the same route day after day, with your headphones, newspaper, and cup of coffee, you are actually *more* vulnerable.

Public Transportation

A potential attacker will see that you aren't paying attention. He or she may have already learned your routine.

Whether you are travelling on a bus, train, airplane, or subway, don't make yourself an easy target. Take precautions.

Try to avoid travelling alone.

Avoid wearing headphones. It is important to hear what is going on around you.

Public Transportation

If someone behaves inappropriately or causes a disturbance on your bus, notify the driver immediately. Most bus companies have a dispatcher, and drivers can have them contact the police if necessary.

If someone sitting next to you makes you feel uncomfortable, move to another seat.

If this person appears to be getting off at your stop, stay on the bus or subway and exit at the next stop.

Public Transportation

If you are routinely harassed by an individual, notify the driver and the police. Change your route and travel time, if possible.

Always be aware of the people around you. Thefts and robberies frequently take place at airports, bus stops, and train and subway stations.

Don't leave personal belongings unattended. Keep them right next to you or in your lap.

Public Transportation

Keep your money, credit cards, and identification on you, preferably in your front pants pocket.

Never count your money in front of others.

When using a pay phone, be aware of the people standing near or behind you. Many thieves will try to obtain your calling card number. They will watch you dial or listen to the numbers you give the operator. This is called "shoulder surfing."

Public Transportation

Make sure your tickets are easily accessible. You should be able to check your gate, departure time, and other information without having to fumble with your purse or baggage. Digging through your bags will only make you vulnerable to pickpockets.

Don't get distracted if someone asks you questions. Thieves often work in groups— one may try to distract you while another takes your purse, briefcase, or luggage.

Don't give out personal information to strangers—such as the name of your hotel—especially if you are travelling alone.

Hotels

If you are travelling alone and need to stop for the night, stay at a safe, clean, reputable hotel.

When you arrive at the hotel, have a bellhop check that there is no one inside your room.

Do not carry too much luggage.

Always keep one hand free.

Keep your hotel door locked with the inside latch.

Don't let strangers into your room.

Before opening your door to employees, check their ID.

Keep your valuables locked in the safe, if one is available.

Hotels

Instead of charging bar drinks and other hotel services to your room, pay for them with cash. This will help prevent strangers from overhearing your name and room number.

When taking a taxi, choose a reputable company.

Have an idea where you are going and how far away it is. If you don't know, ask a hotel employee.

ON THE ROAD

Driving should not be stressful or dangerous, but women travelling alone need to be particularly attentive to their surroundings.

Know where you are going.

Bring a map in case you get lost.

Bring extra gas money, change for phone calls, and a credit card for emergencies.

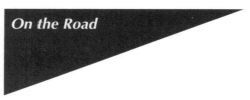

On the Road

Carry a cellular phone with you at all times.

Keep a first aid kit, extra clothing, and blankets in your trunk.

Make sure maps and car rental agreements are out of sight when you're not using them.

Don't pull over on side streets or in unlighted areas.

If you are lost, stop in a busy area to ask for directions or look at a map.

On the Road

Stay on main roads when stopping for food or gas.

Never pull over to sleep on the side of the road. Find a reputable hotel located on a main road.

Park in well-lighted areas close to buildings and walkways.

Do not tell strangers you are travelling alone.

On the Road

Never give a ride to a stranger.

If a stranger has car trouble or needs assistance, you can drive to the nearest pay phone or call for help on your cellular phone.

If you are being followed, go to the nearest business and call the police.

If someone intentionally hits your vehicle or tries to push you off the road:

On the Road

- Ignore the damage—just keep driving.
- Call the police immediately on your cellular phone.
- Go to the nearest business, police station, or fire station to get help.
- Try to remember the last exit or landmark you passed when the car hit you.
- Obtain the license plate number, make, model, and color of the vehicle.
- Note the driver's description and how many passengers were in the car.

If Your Car Breaks Down

Always carry the number for a roadside assistance service that can tow your car or change a flat tire, no matter where you are.

If your vehicle stalls or breaks down, you will need to know your location. The police will not automatically know where you are if you dial 911 from your cellular phone.

*If Your Car
Breaks Down*

If your vehicle breaks down in the city, look for street signs to identify your location.

If you stall on the freeway, try to see the exit ahead of you or remember the last exit you passed. Look for mile markers.

Some states have telephones on the highway that will automatically connect you to highway patrol or roadside assistance.

**If Your Car
Breaks Down**

If you don't have access to a phone, stay in your vehicle until help arrives.

If someone stops to help you, do not accept a ride to a telephone. Ask this individual to call the police for you.

If you must accept a ride, use your intuition. If one person makes you feel uncomfortable, wait for someone else to come along.

If Your Car Breaks Down

Once you get inside a stranger's vehicle, tell him or her that someone is expecting you and will probably start looking for you if you don't call as soon as possible.

If the stranger believes that your family or the police are looking for you, it could deter a potential kidnapping.

Do not give the stranger personal information or details about where you are going.

*If Your Car
Breaks Down*

If the stranger becomes aggressive, look for an opportunity to get out of the vehicle and away from danger.

Say that you aren't feeling well and ask the stranger to pull over to the curb because you need to vomit. This may prevent a potential attack.

Road Rage

Violence on the road is becoming more and more common. Many confrontations have ended in serious injury or death.

You can't control the other drivers on the road, but you *can* control your response to drivers who try to provoke you.

Always stay calm while driving.

Do not tailgate, flash your headlights, slam on your brakes, or make obscene gestures. These will only enrage the other driver, putting your safety at risk.

Road Rage

If someone tailgates your car, pull over to let him or her pass.

Avoid eye contact with other drivers; don't even look toward another vehicle, if you can help it.

Never respond to a challenge.

If a driver tries to force or coerce you off the road, keep moving. Use your cellular phone to call the police, or drive to a safe place where other people can assist you.

Road Rage

If you are involved in an accident and the other driver behaves in a threatening manner, stay in your locked vehicle until help arrives.

If the driver becomes violent and you feel your safety is at risk, drive to a safe place and call the police.

Try to obtain the license plate number of the vehicle, as well as a physical description of the driver.

Attackers Impersonating Police Officers

Criminals are becoming more creative—and even more dangerous—when it comes to seeking out victims.

In some instances, attackers have actually dressed as police officers and stopped unsuspecting women who were travelling alone.

Although incidents like these are rare, you should always be cautious. If you are pulled over by someone who appears to be a police officer, look for the following:

Attackers Impersonating Police Officers

Is the Officer in a Marked Squad Car?

If a police officer stops you for a traffic violation, he or she will *usually* be in a marked patrol car.

A marked car will *always* have red (or red and blue) lights on top.

The license plate will probably read POLICE.

**Attackers Impersonating
Police Officers**

If the officer is in an unmarked car, look for red lights, or a combination of red and blue lights.

If you only see blue lights (or no lights at all), the driver is not a legitimate police officer.

Drive away immediately and report the incident to the police.

Attackers Impersonating Police Officers

Is the Officer Wearing a Uniform?

Whether the police officer is in a marked or unmarked squad car, he or she will *usually* be wearing a uniform with a badge or patch on the shirt or jacket.

The patch should read "highway patrol" or list the city or county you are in.

If the individual is not wearing a uniform or you cannot see the patch, ask for identification.

If the individual refuses or becomes irate, drive to the nearest business to get help.

AFTER AN ATTACK

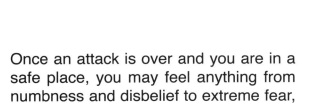

Once an attack is over and you are in a safe place, you may feel anything from numbness and disbelief to extreme fear, anxiety, and disorganization.

You might feel angry, guilty, fearful, depressed, and humiliated.

If you have been injured, you may be in physical pain as well.

After notifying the police, it is important to get medical treatment immediately, even if you have no obvious injuries.

It is equally important to surround yourself with friends, family, or counselors who can comfort and support you.

Even minor attacks can have an enormous emotional impact, so be gentle with yourself in the days and weeks that follow. No matter what you may think, you are not to blame.

The fact that you survived the attack is a testimony to your strength. Use this strength to recover from the assault and regain control of your life.

A WORD ABOUT WEAPONS

A Word about Weapons

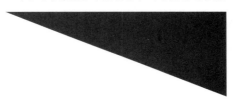

Many things can be used as a weapon—
a gun, knife, baseball bat, stick, flash-
light, fist, mace, even a set of keys.

An attacker might use any of these, and
so can you.

If you are attacked, reach for anything
you can use as a weapon. Be creative.

If you choose to carry a weapon, whether
it be mace in your purse or a gun in your
house, make sure you are trained, expe-
rienced, and psychologically prepared to
use it.

A Word about Weapons

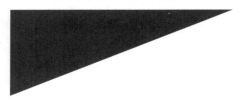

A moment's hesitation may give an attacker enough time to disarm you.

Be sure your weapon is accessible. If you are attacked, and your mace is in your purse, you may not be able to get to it in time.

Remember, too, that any weapon you carry has the potential to be used against you.

Mace

Although mace may startle an attacker, perhaps giving you enough time to get away, the chemical doesn't work on everyone.

Spraying mace on someone who is intoxicated or on drugs might only agitate him or her further.

Mace might also prevent you from escaping an attack. Once sprayed, the chemical will linger in the air. If you come in contact with it, you may not be able to see or function well enough to get away.

Personal Alarms

Many women carry a hand-held screech alarm. While a personal alarm is not an actual weapon, it does have certain advantages.

Screech alarms are loud enough to call attention to yourself and your attacker. This makes most attackers uncomfortable, and they may be less willing to follow through with their assault.

Unlike mace, an alarm will not prevent you from escaping. Furthermore, it cannot be used against you.

Self-Defense

Some women choose self-defense as a personal protection strategy.

There are several different ways to strike an attacker, but unless you are trained properly and practice the techniques repeatedly, you might forget what to do in a crisis.

If you are in a situation where you must defend yourself, don't hold back. Do whatever you can to get away.

Distract your attacker by aiming at vulnerable areas on the body.

- Bite your attacker on the hand, hard.
- Kick him or her in the groin or shins.
- Strike the Adam's apple with the side of your hand.
- Poke the eyes with your fingers.
- Use the heel of your hand to come up sharply underneath his or her nose.

These strikes may help you escape an attacker, but they are not always effective. Do not rely on them to protect yourself.

While weapons and martial arts training might be an option for some women, they are certainly not essential to a woman's safety.

You already have everything you need to protect yourself. Use your experience and common sense, practice what you have learned, and be aware of your surroundings. Remember, you are your best defense against crime.

Women don't have to be stronger than their attackers, just smarter.

Important Phone Numbers

Emergency_____911_____

Police_____

Fire_____

Ambulance_____

Taxi_____

Roadside Assistance_____

Bank_____

Credit Card Company_____

Insurance Company_____

Security

Apartment_____

Work_____

Campus_____

Escort

Work_____

Campus_____

Crisis Lines

Sexual Assault_____

Domestic Violence_____

Janeé Harteau is an Investigator in the Organized Crime Unit of the Minneapolis Police Department.

Holly Keegel is an officer in the Safe Unit of the Minneapolis Police Department. She specializes in crime prevention.

With over twenty years combined law enforcement experience, Harteau and Keegel are the founders of Women's Street Survival, Inc. They are available for speaking engagements and group training seminars. For more information, contact SafeWomen@aol.com.

Harteau and Keegel live in the Twin Cities, Minnesota.